THE COMPREHENSIVE HYSTERECTOMY COOKBOOK:

Eating for Healing

Contents

1. INTRODUCTION

The introduction of "The Comprehensive Hysterectomy Cookbook: Eating for Healing" serves as a warm welcome and an overview of the cookbook's purpose and contents. It's an opportunity to connect with readers, establish the context of the book and highlight its importance in the journey of recovery post-hysterectomy. Here's a possible outline for the introduction:

1. Welcoming Readers: Offer a warm greeting and express gratitude to readers for choosing the cookbook as a resource during their recovery journey.

2. The Significance of Nutrition in Recovery: Emphasize the critical role of nutrition in supporting the healing process after a hysterectomy, explaining how the right diet can aid in restoring energy, managing pain and promoting overall well-being.

3. Purpose of the Cookbook: Clearly define the purpose and goals of the cookbook, emphasizing its focus on providing delicious, nutritious and easy-to-prepare recipes tailored to support the specific nutritional needs of individuals recovering from a hysterectomy.

4. Empowerment through Food: Discuss how the cookbook aims to empower readers to take an active role in

their recovery journey by making informed and nourishing food choices, thereby enhancing their overall wellness and quality of life.

5. Support and Guidance: Reassure readers that the cookbook is not just a collection of recipes but also a comprehensive guide filled with practical tips, expert advice and emotional support to help them navigate the challenges and changes that come with the recovery process.

6. A Note on Personal Journey: Share a brief personal story or anecdote to establish a connection with readers and to create a sense of empathy and understanding.

7. How to Use This Cookbook: Provide a brief guide on how readers can effectively navigate the cookbook, including an explanation of the structure, layout and key sections, encouraging them to use it as a tool for creating a balanced and nourishing meal plan.

By setting the tone for the cookbook and highlighting its purpose, you can engage readers from the outset, motivating them to embark on a healing journey supported by nutritious and delicious meals.

Understanding Hysterectomy: What to Expect

Understanding what to expect from a hysterectomy is crucial for anyone preparing for this surgical procedure. A hysterectomy involves the removal of a woman's uterus and possibly other reproductive organs and it can have significant physical and emotional impacts. Here are some key points to consider:

1. Explanation of the Procedure: Describe the surgical process involved in a hysterectomy, including the different types of hysterectomy (total, partial, radical) and the reasons why it may be recommended by a healthcare provider.

2. Preoperative Preparation: Discuss the steps involved in preparing for a hysterectomy, which may include pre-surgery tests, dietary adjustments and lifestyle changes.

3. Recovery Period: Explain the typical recovery timeline and what patients can expect in terms of physical discomfort, pain management and limitations on activities during the healing process.

4. Potential Risks and Complications: Provide an overview of potential risks associated with the surgery, such as infection, bleeding and potential long-term effects, including changes in hormonal balance.

5. Emotional and Psychological Impact: Discuss the potential emotional effects of undergoing a hysterectomy, including the impact on body image, fertility concerns and coping strategies for managing emotional challenges.

6. Post-Surgery Care: Offer insights into the importance of follow-up appointments, medication management and lifestyle adjustments post-surgery to ensure a smooth recovery and minimize potential complications.

7. Long-Term Implications: Provide information on the potential long-term implications of a hysterectomy, including its impact on sexual health, bone health and overall well-being.

It's essential to provide a comprehensive understanding of the procedure, recovery and long-term implications to help readers feel informed and prepared for the journey ahead. Moreover, addressing the emotional and psychological aspects can offer significant support for individuals navigating the emotional challenges associated with this surgery.

Importance of Nutrition in Recovery

In the context of a hysterectomy, proper nutrition plays a crucial role in supporting the body's healing process and overall well-being. In the section discussing the importance of nutrition in recovery, consider including the following points:

1. Nourishing the Healing Process: Explain how a well-balanced and nutrient-rich diet can provide the body with the essential building blocks it needs to repair tissues, promote wound healing and regain strength after surgery.

2. Boosting Energy Levels: Emphasize how the right combination of carbohydrates, proteins and healthy fats can help replenish energy levels, combat fatigue and support a faster recovery, enabling individuals to resume daily activities with more vitality.

3. Supporting Immune Function: Discuss how certain nutrients, such as vitamins A, C and E, along with zinc and other immune-boosting elements, can strengthen the immune system, helping to prevent infections and other complications during the recovery period.

4. Managing Inflammation and Pain: Highlight the anti-inflammatory properties of specific foods and nutrients, such as omega-3 fatty acids, antioxidants and certain herbs

and spices, which can help reduce inflammation and alleviate post-surgery discomfort.

5. Promoting Bowel Health: Discuss the importance of a diet rich in fiber and probiotics to maintain healthy digestion and regular bowel movements, thereby preventing constipation and other gastrointestinal issues that may arise during recovery.

6. Enhancing Emotional Well-being: Address the connection between nutrition and emotional health, emphasizing how consuming a balanced diet can positively impact mood, reduce stress and contribute to an overall sense of well-being during the recovery process.

7. Maintaining Hormonal Balance: Explain how certain foods and nutrients can help regulate hormone levels, managing any hormonal fluctuations that may occur post-hysterectomy and supporting hormonal balance for long-term well-being.

By illustrating the multifaceted role of nutrition in the recovery process, readers can gain a comprehensive understanding of how their dietary choices can directly impact their physical and emotional healing post-hysterectomy. This knowledge can empower them to make informed food choices that will support their journey toward a smoother and more effective recovery.

2. PREPARING FOR SURGERY

Preparing for a hysterectomy involves various aspects that extend beyond dietary considerations. In your cookbook, you can offer comprehensive guidance on preparing for surgery. Here are some key points to include:

1. Preoperative Consultation: Explain the significance of meeting with the healthcare team and the surgeon to discuss the details of the surgery, including the procedure, potential risks and expected outcomes.

2. Preparing the Home Environment: Provide tips on preparing the home for post-surgery recovery, such as creating a comfortable resting area, arranging for assistance with daily tasks and stocking up on essential supplies and groceries.

3. Medication Management: Offer guidance on managing preexisting medications, including any necessary adjustments or restrictions, as well as instructions for any new medications prescribed specifically for the surgery.

4. Preoperative Tests and Screenings: Explain the importance of undergoing any necessary preoperative tests and screenings to ensure that the patient is in optimal health for the surgery. This may include blood tests, imaging scans and other diagnostic procedures.

5. Lifestyle Adjustments: Discuss the importance of making certain lifestyle adjustments before the surgery, such as quitting smoking, reducing alcohol consumption and engaging in light physical activities as recommended by the healthcare provider.

6. Emotional Preparation: Address the emotional aspect of preparing for surgery, including the potential anxieties and fears that may arise. Offer coping strategies and emotional support resources to help individuals manage their emotional well-being during this challenging time.

7. Clearing Doubts and Concerns: Encourage readers to communicate openly with their healthcare providers and address any doubts or concerns they may have about the surgery, the recovery process, or any other related aspects.

By providing comprehensive guidance on how to prepare for the surgery, both physically and emotionally, you can empower readers to approach their hysterectomy with confidence and a sense of preparedness. This proactive approach can contribute to a smoother and more comfortable experience throughout the entire surgical process.

Preoperative Diet Tips

Before undergoing a hysterectomy, it is essential to focus on maintaining a healthy diet to optimize your overall well-being and prepare your body for the surgery. Here are some preoperative diet tips to include in your cookbook:

1. Hydration is Key: Emphasize the importance of staying well-hydrated by consuming an adequate amount of water and other hydrating fluids. Encourage the intake of water-rich foods such as fruits and vegetables to support hydration.

2. Balanced Nutrition: Provide guidance on maintaining a well-balanced diet rich in essential nutrients, including a variety of fruits, vegetables, whole grains, lean proteins and healthy fats. Highlight the importance of incorporating a diverse range of foods to ensure the intake of essential vitamins and minerals.

3. Limit Processed Foods: Suggest minimizing the consumption of processed and high-sodium foods, as these can contribute to bloating and water retention. Encourage readers to opt for whole, natural foods to support overall health and well-being.

4. Fiber Intake: Recommend incorporating high-fiber foods such as whole grains, legumes and fresh fruits and

vegetables to promote regular bowel movements and prevent constipation, which can be exacerbated during the postoperative recovery phase.

5. Reduce Alcohol and Caffeine: Advise limiting the intake of alcohol and caffeine to support overall hydration and minimize any potential negative impacts on the body's preoperative condition.

6. Discuss Supplements: Consider discussing the potential benefits of specific supplements, such as iron or vitamin D, depending on individual needs and deficiencies. However, it is crucial to consult a healthcare provider before initiating any new supplements.

7. Consult with a Healthcare Provider: Stress the importance of consulting with a healthcare provider or a registered dietitian to develop a personalized preoperative diet plan that addresses individual needs and health conditions.

Encouraging readers to adopt these preoperative diet tips can help them prepare their bodies for surgery, potentially reducing the risk of complications and supporting a smoother recovery process.

Hydration and Its Role in Recovery

Proper hydration is crucial for the body's overall functioning, especially during the recovery period following a hysterectomy. In your cookbook, you can provide valuable insights into the role of hydration in the recovery process. Consider including the following points:

1. Importance of Hydration: Emphasize the significance of maintaining adequate hydration levels to support various bodily functions, including the transport of nutrients, elimination of waste products and regulation of body temperature.

2. Fluid Balance and Wound Healing: Explain how proper hydration can facilitate the healing of surgical incisions and promote tissue regeneration, thereby reducing the risk of complications and expediting the recovery process.

3. Management of Medications: Discuss how sufficient hydration can aid in the effective absorption and distribution of medications prescribed during the recovery phase, ensuring their optimal efficacy and promoting a smoother recovery trajectory.

4. Prevention of Constipation: Highlight how adequate fluid intake can prevent constipation, a common postoperative issue, by softening the stool and facilitating

its passage, thus reducing discomfort and promoting gastrointestinal health.

5. Support for Vital Organs: Illustrate how hydration supports the proper functioning of vital organs, including the kidneys and the bladder, thereby reducing the risk of urinary tract infections and other complications that may arise during the recovery period.

6. Optimal Hydration Sources: Provide guidance on the best sources of hydration, including water, herbal teas, clear broths and hydrating fruits and vegetables, while advising against excessive consumption of sugary or caffeinated beverages that can potentially contribute to dehydration.

7. Monitoring Hydration Levels: Recommend monitoring hydration levels by observing urine color and frequency and encourage readers to maintain a consistent intake of fluids throughout the day to ensure adequate hydration.

By educating readers on the importance of hydration and its direct impact on the recovery process, you can empower them to prioritize their fluid intake and actively participate in their own healing journey following a hysterectomy.

3. POST-SURGERY NUTRITION BASICS

After undergoing a hysterectomy, maintaining proper nutrition is vital for supporting the body's healing process and promoting overall well-being. In the section on post-surgery nutrition basics, consider including the following points in your cookbook:

1. Soft and Easily Digestible Foods: Recommend incorporating soft and easily digestible foods such as soups, broths and cooked vegetables to ease digestion and minimize discomfort during the initial postoperative period.

2. Protein-Rich Foods: Emphasize the importance of consuming adequate amounts of protein to support tissue repair and promote muscle strength. Suggest easily digestible protein sources such as lean meats, fish, eggs and legumes.

3. Essential Nutrients for Healing: Highlight the significance of essential nutrients such as vitamins A, C, D and E, as well as minerals like zinc and iron, in supporting the body's immune function and facilitating the healing of surgical wounds.

4. Anti-Inflammatory Foods: Recommend incorporating anti-inflammatory foods such as fatty fish, nuts, seeds and

leafy greens to help reduce postoperative inflammation and alleviate discomfort.

5. Fiber-Rich Foods: Encourage the gradual introduction of fiber-rich foods to promote healthy digestion and prevent constipation. Recommend incorporating fruits, vegetables, whole grains and legumes to support regular bowel movements.

6. Hydration: Reinforce the importance of maintaining adequate hydration post-surgery, as it is essential for promoting wound healing, supporting organ function and aiding in the elimination of medications and toxins from the body.

7. Small, Frequent Meals: Suggest consuming small, frequent meals throughout the day to avoid gastrointestinal discomfort and support the body's ability to absorb nutrients efficiently during the recovery period.

8. Meal Preparation Tips: Provide practical meal preparation tips, such as using herbs and spices to add flavor without excessive salt, cooking methods that promote easy digestion and portion control to prevent overeating and digestive discomfort.

By emphasizing these post-surgery nutrition basics, you can guide readers in making informed dietary choices that will support their recovery, minimize discomfort and contribute to an overall smoother healing process following a hysterectomy.

The Healing Power of Nutrients

In the context of post-hysterectomy recovery, it is essential to highlight the healing power of specific nutrients. In your cookbook, you can educate readers about the key nutrients that play a crucial role in supporting the body's healing process. Consider including the following information:

1. Protein for Tissue Repair: Explain how protein is essential for the repair and regeneration of tissues, emphasizing its role in wound healing and the maintenance of muscle mass. Provide information on protein-rich foods that can be incorporated into the diet post-surgery.

2. Vitamins for Immune Support: Discuss the importance of vitamins, particularly vitamin C and vitamin A, in supporting the immune system and promoting the body's defense against infections. Highlight specific foods that are rich in these vitamins and easy to incorporate into meals.

3. Minerals for Bone Health: Highlight the significance of minerals such as calcium and magnesium in maintaining bone health, which is especially crucial for women post-hysterectomy. Provide information on nutrient-dense foods that can help support bone strength and density.

4. Omega-3 Fatty Acids for Inflammation: Explain how omega-3 fatty acids possess anti-inflammatory properties

that can help reduce postoperative inflammation and support overall healing. Recommend dietary sources of omega-3 fatty acids, such as fatty fish, flaxseeds and walnuts.

5. Antioxidants for Tissue Regeneration: Discuss the role of antioxidants in promoting tissue regeneration and protecting cells from oxidative stress, which can aid in the healing of surgical wounds. Highlight antioxidant-rich foods such as berries, leafy greens and colorful vegetables.

6. Fiber for Digestive Health: Emphasize the importance of dietary fiber in maintaining healthy digestion and preventing constipation, which is a common postoperative concern. Recommend fiber-rich foods such as whole grains, fruits, vegetables and legumes.

7. Hydration for Overall Well-being: Reinforce the importance of staying adequately hydrated to support the body's natural healing processes, maintain organ function and facilitate the elimination of toxins. Provide tips on incorporating hydrating foods and beverages into the daily diet.

By educating readers about the healing properties of these essential nutrients, you can empower them to make informed dietary choices that will facilitate a smoother and more effective recovery following a hysterectomy.

Managing Digestive Challenges

After a hysterectomy, many individuals may experience digestive challenges, which can impact their overall well-being and comfort during the recovery period. In your cookbook, you can offer valuable guidance on managing these digestive challenges. Consider including the following points:

1. Introduction to Digestive Challenges: Provide an overview of common digestive issues that may arise post-hysterectomy, such as constipation, bloating and changes in bowel habits and explain the potential reasons behind these challenges.

2. Importance of Fiber Intake: Highlight the importance of consuming an adequate amount of dietary fiber to support healthy digestion and prevent constipation. Recommend fiber-rich foods such as whole grains, fruits, vegetables and legumes to help regulate bowel movements.

3. Hydration for Digestive Health: Emphasize the role of hydration in maintaining healthy digestion and preventing constipation. Encourage readers to consume an adequate amount of water and hydrating fluids throughout the day to support bowel regularity.

4. Gentle Digestive Foods: Recommend incorporating easily digestible foods such as soups, broths, cooked vegetables and soft fruits to minimize digestive discomfort and facilitate the digestion process during the initial recovery phase.

5. Probiotics for Gut Health: Discuss the potential benefits of incorporating probiotic-rich foods or supplements to support gut health and promote a healthy balance of gut bacteria, which can aid in maintaining regular bowel movements.

6. Slow and Mindful Eating: Encourage readers to practice mindful eating and chew their food thoroughly to support proper digestion and prevent digestive discomfort, such as bloating and indigestion.

7. Consultation with a Healthcare Provider: Stress the importance of consulting with a healthcare provider or a registered dietitian if individuals experience persistent or severe digestive challenges, as this may require personalized dietary or medical interventions.

By addressing the management of digestive challenges, you can provide readers with practical strategies to promote digestive health and enhance their overall comfort and well-being during the recovery period following a hysterectomy.

4. EASY-TO-DIGEST RECIPES FOR THE INITIAL DAYS

During the initial days post-hysterectomy, it is essential to consume easily digestible foods that are gentle on the stomach and promote a smooth recovery. In your cookbook, consider including a section on easy-to-digest recipes specifically tailored for this phase. Here are some ideas for such recipes:

1. Nourishing Chicken and Vegetable Broth:

   - A simple broth made with lean chicken, carrots, celery and gentle herbs, simmered to create a flavorful and easily digestible base.

2. Creamy Butternut Squash Soup:

   - A smooth and creamy soup made with butternut squash, low-fat milk and a touch of nutmeg, providing comforting warmth and essential nutrients.

3. Soft Scrambled Eggs with Spinach:

   - Light and fluffy scrambled eggs blended with sautéed spinach, providing a protein-rich and easily digestible option packed with essential nutrients.

4. Mashed Sweet Potatoes with a Hint of Cinnamon:

- Soft and creamy mashed sweet potatoes seasoned with a hint of cinnamon, offering a naturally sweet and easily digestible source of carbohydrates and vitamins.

5. Tender Baked Salmon with Steamed Asparagus:

- Delicately baked salmon fillets served with lightly steamed asparagus, providing a soft and easily digestible source of protein and essential omega-3 fatty acids.

6. Smooth Banana and Yogurt Blend:

- A creamy blend of ripe bananas and probiotic-rich yogurt, offering a gentle and easily digestible option packed with essential nutrients and beneficial bacteria.

7. Simple Rice Congee with Ginger:

- A comforting bowl of rice congee seasoned with fresh ginger, offering a soothing and easily digestible option that provides essential carbohydrates and warmth.

8. Delicate Fruit Compote:

- A mixture of stewed apples, pears and a hint of cinnamon, offering a gentle and easily digestible option packed with natural sweetness and essential vitamins.

These easy-to-digest recipes can help readers navigate the initial days following a hysterectomy, providing nourishing and comforting options that support the recovery process and minimize digestive discomfort.

Nourishing Soups and Broths

Certainly, here are some nourishing soup and broth ideas that can provide comfort and essential nutrients during the recovery period post-hysterectomy:

1. Healing Chicken and Vegetable Broth:

   - A comforting broth made with tender chicken, carrots, celery, onions and a blend of fragrant herbs, simmered to perfection for a nourishing and flavorful base.

2. Creamy Mushroom Soup:

   - A rich and creamy soup featuring a medley of mushrooms, onions, garlic and thyme, blended to a smooth consistency for a comforting and nourishing option.

3. Lentil and Vegetable Soup:

   - A hearty and nutritious soup combining lentils, tomatoes, carrots and spinach, seasoned with aromatic herbs and spices to create a satisfying and protein-rich meal.

4. Nourishing Bone Broth:

   - A wholesome bone broth infused with marrow bones, aromatic vegetables and a hint of apple cider vinegar, simmered for an extended period to extract valuable nutrients and collagen.

5. Comforting Tomato Basil Soup:

   - A classic tomato soup with a twist of fresh basil, garlic and a touch of cream for a soothing and nourishing option that is both flavorful and comforting.

6. Velvety Butternut Squash Soup:

   - A smooth and velvety soup made with roasted butternut squash, onions and warming spices, offering a nourishing and comforting option rich in vitamins and minerals.

7. Vegetable and Barley Broth:

   - A hearty and wholesome broth featuring barley, an array of seasonal vegetables and a blend of aromatic herbs, providing a nourishing and filling option for a comforting meal.

8. Nutrient-Packed Minestrone Soup:

   - A robust and flavorful minestrone soup filled with a variety of vegetables, beans and pasta, offering a nourishing and satisfying option rich in fiber and essential nutrients.

These nourishing soup and broth recipes can provide warmth, comfort and essential nutrients, supporting the recovery process and promoting overall well-being following a hysterectomy.

Soft and Gentle Protein Options

Certainly, during the recovery period after a hysterectomy, it's important to consume soft and gentle protein options that are easy to digest. Here are some protein-rich yet gentle options to consider for your cookbook:

1. Tender Shredded Chicken:

   - Slow-cooked and tender shredded chicken seasoned with mild herbs and spices, providing a soft and easily digestible protein option.

2. Flaky Baked White Fish:

   - Delicately baked white fish such as tilapia or cod, seasoned with a light lemon and herb marinade, offering a gentle and protein-rich option that is easy on the stomach.

3. Silken Tofu Scramble:

   - Soft and silken tofu scrambled with gentle seasoning and fresh herbs, providing a plant-based and easily digestible protein option that is rich in essential nutrients.

4. Poached Eggs:

   - Softly poached eggs served with a sprinkle of herbs or a touch of mild sauce, offering a gentle and protein-packed option that is easy to prepare and digest.

5. Mashed Chickpea Salad:

- Creamy and mashed chickpea salad blended with light dressing, chopped vegetables and herbs, providing a soft and easily digestible plant-based protein option.

6. Smooth Nut Butter:

- Smooth and creamy nut butter, such as almond or cashew butter, served with soft bread or crackers, offering a protein-rich and easily digestible option that is also rich in healthy fats.

7. Cottage Cheese with Fruit:

- Soft and mild cottage cheese served with a side of fresh, ripe fruits, offering a gentle and protein-packed option that is also rich in essential vitamins and minerals.

8. Yogurt Parfait:

- Creamy and soft yogurt layered with fresh fruits, nuts and a touch of honey, providing a protein-rich and easily digestible option that is also rich in probiotics.

These soft and gentle protein options can help provide essential nutrients and support the recovery process following a hysterectomy, ensuring a balanced and nourishing diet during this sensitive period.

5. INCORPORATING ESSENTIAL NUTRIENTS

Incorporating essential nutrients is crucial for supporting the body's healing process and overall well-being post-hysterectomy. Here are some key nutrients to focus on and ideas on how to incorporate them into the diet:

1. Protein:

   - Include lean meats, poultry, fish, eggs, dairy, legumes and plant-based protein sources like tofu and tempeh in meals.

   - Prepare protein-rich smoothies with ingredients like Greek yogurt, nut butter and protein powder for a convenient and nourishing option.

2. Calcium and Vitamin D:

   - Incorporate dairy products, fortified plant-based milk, leafy greens and fortified cereals to support bone health.

   - Create nutrient-rich salads with spinach, kale and collard greens, combined with calcium-fortified tofu or canned fish with edible bones like sardines.

3. Iron:

   - Include iron-rich foods such as lean red meat, poultry, fish, legumes and fortified cereals to help replenish iron stores and prevent anemia.

- Prepare meals with ingredients like spinach, lentils and beans to boost iron intake and support overall energy levels.

4. Vitamin C:

- Pair iron-rich foods with vitamin C sources like citrus fruits, strawberries, bell peppers and broccoli to enhance iron absorption.

- Create refreshing fruit salads or vegetable stir-fries incorporating a variety of colorful, vitamin C-rich produce.

5. Fiber:

- Incorporate whole grains, fruits, vegetables, nuts and seeds to promote healthy digestion and prevent constipation.

- Prepare nutrient-dense salads with a mix of leafy greens, colorful vegetables and fiber-rich additions like quinoa, nuts and beans.

6. Healthy Fats:

- Include sources of healthy fats such as avocados, nuts, seeds, olive oil and fatty fish to support overall health and provide essential fatty acids.

- Create flavorful and nutritious salads drizzled with homemade olive oil-based dressings or incorporate avocado into smoothies for a creamy and nourishing texture.

By emphasizing the incorporation of these essential nutrients into daily meals, you can provide readers with practical strategies to support their recovery and promote overall well-being following a hysterectomy.

Vitamins and Minerals for Recovery

In the post-hysterectomy recovery period, it's essential to focus on incorporating a variety of vitamins and minerals into the diet to support overall healing and well-being. Here are some key vitamins and minerals to emphasize, along with ideas on how to include them in meals:

1. Vitamin A:

  - Incorporate foods such as sweet potatoes, carrots, dark leafy greens and bell peppers into salads, soups, or as side dishes to support immune function and promote tissue repair.

2. Vitamin C:

  - Include citrus fruits, strawberries, kiwi and tomatoes in salads, smoothies, or as refreshing snacks to support collagen formation and boost the immune system.

3. Vitamin D:

- Choose vitamin D-fortified dairy or plant-based milk, incorporate fatty fish like salmon or mackerel and spend time outdoors in sunlight to support bone health and immune function.

4. Vitamin E:

- Use oils such as sunflower, safflower and wheat germ oil in dressings or marinades and incorporate nuts, seeds and spinach into meals to promote tissue healing and protect cells from damage.

5. B vitamins:

- Include whole grains, eggs, dairy, legumes and leafy greens in meals to support energy production and nervous system function, helping to reduce fatigue and promote overall well-being.

6. Calcium:

- Incorporate dairy products, fortified plant-based milk, tofu and leafy greens into meals to support bone health and muscle function.

7. Iron:

- Choose iron-rich foods such as lean meats, poultry, fish, legumes and fortified cereals to help replenish iron stores and prevent anemia.

8. Magnesium:

- Incorporate nuts, seeds, whole grains, legumes and leafy greens into meals to support muscle and nerve function and promote overall relaxation and well-being.

By emphasizing the importance of incorporating a variety of vitamins and minerals into meals, you can help readers create a well-rounded and nourishing diet that supports their recovery and overall health after a hysterectomy.

Creating Balanced Meals

Creating balanced meals is essential for promoting overall well-being and supporting the recovery process following a hysterectomy. Here are some guidelines to help readers create well-rounded and nourishing meals:

1. Incorporate a Variety of Food Groups: Include a mix of fruits, vegetables, whole grains, lean proteins and healthy fats in each meal to ensure a diverse range of nutrients.

2. Prioritize Colorful Produce: Encourage the inclusion of a variety of colorful fruits and vegetables to provide a wide array of vitamins, minerals and antioxidants that support overall health and healing.

3. Include Lean Proteins: Incorporate lean protein sources such as poultry, fish, legumes and tofu to support tissue repair and promote muscle strength.

4. Opt for Whole Grains: Choose whole grains like brown rice, quinoa and whole wheat pasta to provide fiber, vitamins and minerals that support digestion and overall health.

5. Incorporate Healthy Fats: Include sources of healthy fats such as avocados, nuts, seeds and olive oil to support heart health and provide essential fatty acids.

6. Mindful Portion Control: Encourage mindful portion control to prevent overeating and support digestion, allowing the body to efficiently absorb nutrients without causing discomfort.

7. Hydration with Nutrient-Rich Beverages: Recommend hydrating with water, herbal teas and nutrient-rich smoothies to support overall hydration and provide additional vitamins and minerals.

8. Experiment with Herbs and Spices: Encourage the use of herbs and spices to add flavor and variety to meals without relying on excessive salt or added sugars.

9. Balance Macronutrients: Ensure each meal contains a balance of carbohydrates, proteins and healthy fats to provide sustained energy and support overall bodily functions.

By guiding readers on how to create balanced meals, you can empower them to make informed and nourishing food choices that support their recovery and promote overall well-being after a hysterectomy.

6. BUILDING STRENGTH AND ENERGY

Building strength and energy is essential during the recovery period following a hysterectomy. Consider including the following tips and suggestions in your cookbook to help readers effectively boost their strength and energy levels:

1. Protein-Packed Dishes: Provide recipes rich in lean proteins such as chicken, fish, legumes and tofu to support muscle repair and growth, promoting overall strength and vitality.

2. Energizing Smoothies and Juices: Offer recipes for nutrient-dense smoothies and juices that incorporate fruits, vegetables and protein sources such as Greek yogurt or protein powder to provide a quick and easily digestible source of energy.

3. Healthy Carbohydrates: Encourage the consumption of complex carbohydrates like whole grains, sweet potatoes and quinoa, which provide sustained energy and support overall vitality.

4. Vitamin and Mineral-Rich Foods: Highlight the importance of incorporating foods rich in vitamins and minerals, such as leafy greens, citrus fruits and nuts, to support energy production and overall well-being.

5. Hydration for Energy: Emphasize the significance of staying adequately hydrated to maintain energy levels, as dehydration can lead to fatigue and decreased vitality. Encourage the consumption of water, herbal teas and hydrating fruits and vegetables.

6. Balanced Meals and Snacks: Suggest the consumption of balanced meals and snacks throughout the day to maintain stable blood sugar levels and prevent energy fluctuations. Encourage the combination of protein, healthy fats and complex carbohydrates in each meal to promote sustained energy.

7. Light Exercise Recommendations: Provide gentle exercise recommendations approved by a healthcare provider, such as short walks or light stretching, to gradually build strength and energy levels without overexertion.

8. Adequate Rest and Recovery: Stress the importance of allowing the body to rest and recover adequately to

conserve energy and support the healing process, thereby promoting overall well-being and vitality.

By incorporating these strategies, you can empower readers to make informed dietary choices and lifestyle adjustments that will support their journey towards building strength and enhancing energy levels during the recovery period post-hysterectomy.

Protein-Packed Dishes for Recovery

Certainly, incorporating protein-rich dishes into the diet can aid in the recovery process following a hysterectomy. Here are some protein-packed dish ideas for your cookbook:

1. Grilled Lemon Herb Chicken:

   - Tender grilled chicken marinated with a blend of fresh herbs and lemon juice, providing a flavorful and protein-rich main course option.

2. Baked Salmon with Dill and Garlic:

   - Delicate salmon fillets baked with a hint of dill and garlic, offering a soft and protein-packed seafood option that is rich in omega-3 fatty acids.

3. Lentil and Vegetable Stew:

   - Hearty stew featuring lentils, carrots, celery and tomatoes, providing a nourishing and protein-rich plant-based option packed with essential nutrients and fiber.

4. Quinoa and Black Bean Salad:

   - Wholesome salad combining quinoa, black beans, colorful bell peppers and a zesty lime dressing, offering a protein-rich and refreshing option that is also rich in dietary fiber.

5. Tofu Stir-Fry with Mixed Vegetables:

   - Tofu stir-fry featuring an array of colorful vegetables, ginger and soy sauce, providing a plant-based and protein-packed option that is both satisfying and nourishing.

6. Greek Yogurt and Berry Parfait:

   - Creamy Greek yogurt layered with a variety of fresh berries and a sprinkle of granola, providing a protein-rich and refreshing option that is also rich in essential vitamins and antioxidants.

7. Egg and Vegetable Frittata:

   - Light and fluffy frittata loaded with a mix of sautéed vegetables and herbs, providing a protein-rich and satisfying option that is easy to prepare and customize.

8. Turkey and Vegetable Skewers:

   - Grilled skewers featuring tender turkey chunks and a colorful array of bell peppers and onions, offering a protein-packed and visually appealing dish that is both flavorful and nourishing.

By incorporating these protein-packed dishes, you can provide readers with a variety of delicious and nourishing options that will support their recovery and promote overall well-being following a hysterectomy.

Energizing Smoothie and Juice Recipes

Certainly, here are some energizing smoothie and juice recipes that can provide a quick and easily digestible source of energy during the recovery period:

Energizing Smoothie Recipes:

1. Tropical Green Smoothie:

   - Blend together spinach, pineapple, mango, banana and a splash of coconut water for a refreshing and nutrient-rich tropical smoothie.

2. Berry Protein Smoothie:

   - Combine mixed berries, Greek yogurt, almond milk and a scoop of protein powder for a satisfying and protein-packed smoothie that promotes muscle recovery.

3. Banana Almond Butter Smoothie:

   - Blend ripe bananas, almond butter, dates and a dash of cinnamon with almond milk for a creamy and energizing smoothie rich in healthy fats and carbohydrates.

4. Green Tea and Mango Smoothie:

- Mix brewed green tea, frozen mango chunks, Greek yogurt and honey for a revitalizing and antioxidant-rich smoothie that provides a gentle energy boost.

Energizing Juice Recipes:

1. Carrot-Apple-Ginger Juice:

- Juice fresh carrots, apples and a hint of ginger for a zesty and vitamin-packed beverage that provides a natural energy boost and supports overall well-being.

2. Citrus-Berry Blast Juice:

- Combine oranges, strawberries and a touch of lemon for a refreshing and vitamin C-rich juice that helps enhance energy levels and supports immune function.

3. Beetroot and Berry Juice:

- Juice beets, mixed berries and a splash of lime for a vibrant and nutrient-dense beverage that promotes natural energy production and supports overall vitality.

4. Cucumber Mint Refresher:

- Juice cucumbers, fresh mint leaves and a squeeze of lime for a hydrating and rejuvenating beverage that helps combat fatigue and promotes hydration.

These energizing smoothie and juice recipes can provide readers with a quick and convenient way to boost their energy levels and support their recovery following a hysterectomy.

7. MANAGING PAIN AND INFLAMMATION THROUGH DIET

Managing pain and inflammation through diet can play a significant role in supporting the recovery process after a hysterectomy. Here are some dietary recommendations to help manage pain and inflammation:

1. Anti-Inflammatory Foods: Encourage the consumption of foods with natural anti-inflammatory properties, such as fatty fish (salmon, mackerel), leafy greens (spinach, kale) and nuts (almonds, walnuts).

2. Healthy Fats: Suggest incorporating healthy fats like avocados, olive oil and nuts, which contain monounsaturated and polyunsaturated fats that can help reduce inflammation and support overall well-being.

3. Colorful Fruits and Vegetables: Recommend including a variety of colorful fruits and vegetables rich in antioxidants, such as berries, cherries, tomatoes and bell peppers, to help combat oxidative stress and reduce inflammation.

4. Herbs and Spices: Highlight the benefits of using herbs and spices with anti-inflammatory properties, such as turmeric, ginger, garlic and cinnamon, to add flavor to meals while promoting natural pain relief and reducing inflammation.

5. Whole Grains: Encourage the consumption of whole grains like brown rice, quinoa and oats, which provide complex carbohydrates and fiber, contributing to stable blood sugar levels and potentially reducing inflammation.

6. Limiting Processed Foods and Sugar: Advise minimizing the intake of processed foods, refined carbohydrates and added sugars, which can contribute to inflammation and potentially exacerbate postoperative pain.

7. Hydration: Emphasize the importance of staying well-hydrated with water, herbal teas and hydrating foods, as proper hydration can help flush out toxins and reduce inflammation.

8. Omega-3 Fatty Acids: Encourage the consumption of foods rich in omega-3 fatty acids, such as chia seeds, flaxseeds and walnuts, or consider supplementing with fish oil, as these can help reduce inflammation and alleviate pain.

By incorporating these dietary strategies into their daily routine, individuals can potentially manage pain and inflammation more effectively, promoting a smoother and more comfortable recovery process following a hysterectomy.

Anti-inflammatory Foods and Recipes

Incorporating anti-inflammatory foods into the diet can be beneficial for managing pain and promoting overall well-being during the recovery period after a hysterectomy. Consider including the following anti-inflammatory foods and recipe ideas in your cookbook:

Anti-Inflammatory Foods:

1. Fatty Fish: Salmon, mackerel and sardines, rich in omega-3 fatty acids that help reduce inflammation and support overall health.

2. Leafy Greens: Spinach, kale and Swiss chard, packed with antioxidants and phytochemicals that combat inflammation and promote wellness.

3. Berries: Blueberries, strawberries and raspberries, abundant in antioxidants and flavonoids that help reduce inflammation and support the immune system.

4. Nuts: Almonds, walnuts and pistachios, high in healthy fats and antioxidants that contribute to reducing inflammation and promoting heart health.

5. Turmeric: A potent anti-inflammatory spice containing curcumin, which may help alleviate pain and reduce inflammation.

6. Olive Oil: A source of monounsaturated fats and antioxidants that can help lower levels of inflammation and support heart health.

Anti-Inflammatory Recipe Ideas:

1. Grilled Salmon with Turmeric:

   - Marinate salmon with turmeric, garlic and lemon juice, then grill to create a flavorful and anti-inflammatory main course.

2. Spinach and Berry Salad:

   - Combine fresh spinach, mixed berries and walnuts, then drizzle with a light olive oil and balsamic vinaigrette to create a refreshing and anti-inflammatory salad.

3. Turmeric Ginger Smoothie:

   - Blend together turmeric, ginger, pineapple and coconut milk for a creamy and anti-inflammatory smoothie packed with flavor and beneficial nutrients.

4. Sautéed Kale with Garlic and Almonds:

- Sauté kale with minced garlic and top with toasted almonds for a simple and nutritious side dish that is both anti-inflammatory and delicious.

5. Mixed Berry Chia Pudding:

- Combine mixed berries with chia seeds and almond milk to create a satisfying and anti-inflammatory pudding that serves as a nutritious breakfast or dessert option.

By incorporating these anti-inflammatory foods and recipes into their diet, individuals can support their recovery and overall well-being following a hysterectomy.

Healthy Fats for Pain Management

Incorporating healthy fats into the diet can play a significant role in managing pain and promoting overall well-being during the recovery period after a hysterectomy. Consider including the following healthy fats and recipe ideas in your cookbook:

Healthy Fats:

1. Avocado: Rich in monounsaturated fats and antioxidants, avocados can help reduce inflammation and support heart health.

2. Olive Oil: A staple of the Mediterranean diet, olive oil is high in monounsaturated fats and has anti-inflammatory properties that can help manage pain.

3. Nuts and Seeds: Almonds, walnuts, chia seeds and flaxseeds are excellent sources of healthy fats, fiber and antioxidants, which can aid in reducing inflammation and promoting overall wellness.

4. Fatty Fish: Salmon, trout and mackerel are rich in omega-3 fatty acids, which have anti-inflammatory properties and can help alleviate pain and support heart health.

5. Coconut: Coconut and coconut oil contain medium-chain triglycerides that can help reduce inflammation and provide a quick source of energy.

Healthy Fat Recipe Ideas:

1. Avocado Toast with Poached Egg:

   - Spread ripe avocado on whole-grain toast and top with a poached egg and a sprinkle of black pepper for a nutritious and pain-relieving breakfast option.

2. Mixed Nut and Seed Trail Mix:

   - Combine almonds, walnuts, chia seeds and dried fruits to create a satisfying and portable snack that is rich in healthy fats and antioxidants.

3. Baked Salmon with Herb and Olive Oil Drizzle:

   - Bake salmon fillets with a drizzle of olive oil and a sprinkle of fresh herbs to create a flavorful and pain-relieving main course.

4. Coconut Curry Chicken:

- Prepare a fragrant coconut curry with chicken, vegetables and aromatic spices to create a nourishing and anti-inflammatory dish that is both comforting and delicious.

5. Chia Seed Pudding with Almond Butter:

- Mix chia seeds with almond milk and top with a dollop of almond butter for a creamy and nutritious dessert that is rich in healthy fats and antioxidants.

By incorporating these healthy fats and recipe ideas into their diet, individuals can support their recovery and overall well-being following a hysterectomy, while managing pain more effectively.

8. REGULATING HORMONES NATURALLY

Regulating hormones naturally can contribute to overall well-being and support the recovery process after a hysterectomy. Consider including the following tips and dietary suggestions in your cookbook to help readers maintain hormone balance:

1. Healthy Fats: Incorporate foods rich in omega-3 fatty acids, such as salmon, chia seeds and walnuts, to support hormone production and balance.

2. Fiber-Rich Foods: Encourage the consumption of fiber-rich foods like whole grains, fruits and vegetables, as they can help regulate hormone levels and promote overall digestive health.

3. Plant-Based Proteins: Include plant-based protein sources such as legumes, tofu and quinoa to support hormone balance and provide essential amino acids for overall wellness.

4. Cruciferous Vegetables: Suggest the consumption of cruciferous vegetables like broccoli, cauliflower and Brussels sprouts, as they contain compounds that can help regulate estrogen levels and promote hormone balance.

5. Flaxseeds: Recommend incorporating ground flaxseeds into meals, as they contain lignans that may help balance hormone levels, particularly estrogen.

6. Probiotic-Rich Foods: Encourage the consumption of probiotic-rich foods like yogurt, kefir and fermented vegetables, as they can help support gut health and indirectly influence hormone balance.

7. Antioxidant-Rich Fruits: Emphasize the importance of consuming antioxidant-rich fruits such as berries, citrus fruits and pomegranates to support overall health and hormonal balance.

8. Herbal Teas: Suggest herbal teas like chamomile, peppermint and ginger, which can have calming effects and help support hormonal balance through their soothing properties.

By incorporating these dietary suggestions into their daily routine, individuals can potentially support hormone regulation and overall well-being following a hysterectomy. It's essential to consult with a healthcare provider for personalized advice and guidance.

Balancing Hormonal Changes Post-Hysterectomy

Balancing hormonal changes post-hysterectomy is crucial for overall well-being and health. Consider including the following strategies in your cookbook to help readers manage hormonal changes effectively:

1. Nutrient-Dense Diet: Emphasize the importance of consuming a balanced diet rich in whole grains, lean proteins, healthy fats and a variety of fruits and vegetables to support overall hormonal balance.

2. Phytoestrogen-Rich Foods: Suggest incorporating foods rich in phytoestrogens such as soy products, flaxseeds and legumes, which may help balance estrogen levels naturally.

3. Stress Management: Include stress-reducing techniques like meditation, deep breathing exercises and gentle yoga to help manage stress, which can impact hormone levels and overall well-being.

4. Regular Exercise: Encourage engaging in regular physical activity such as walking, swimming, or gentle strength training, as exercise can help regulate hormone levels and promote overall health.

5. Adequate Sleep: Stress the importance of getting sufficient and restful sleep to support hormonal balance and overall wellness, as sleep plays a vital role in hormone regulation.

6. Mindful Eating: Encourage mindful eating practices, such as being aware of hunger cues and choosing nutrient-dense, hormone-balancing foods to support overall well-being and health.

7. Hormone-Supporting Herbs: Highlight the benefits of incorporating hormone-supporting herbs such as maca root, black cohosh and chasteberry, which may help regulate hormone levels and alleviate symptoms of hormonal imbalance.

8. Consultation with Healthcare Providers: Stress the importance of consulting healthcare providers, including gynecologists and endocrinologists, for guidance and support in managing hormonal changes post-hysterectomy.

By incorporating these strategies into their daily routines, individuals can potentially manage hormonal changes more effectively and support their overall well-being and health after a hysterectomy. It's essential to consult with healthcare providers for personalized advice and guidance based on individual needs and circumstances.

Foods for Hormonal Stability

Focusing on foods that promote hormonal stability can be beneficial for individuals post-hysterectomy. Consider including the following hormone-stabilizing foods and dietary recommendations in your cookbook:

1. Complex Carbohydrates: Encourage the consumption of whole grains like brown rice, quinoa and oats, which can help stabilize blood sugar levels and support hormonal balance.

2. Healthy Fats: Include sources of healthy fats such as avocados, nuts, seeds and olive oil, which can help support hormone production and overall hormonal stability.

3. Leafy Greens: Suggest incorporating leafy greens like spinach, kale and Swiss chard, which are rich in vitamins and minerals that support hormonal health and balance.

4. Lean Proteins: Encourage the consumption of lean protein sources such as chicken, turkey, fish and legumes, which provide essential amino acids necessary for hormone production and regulation.

5. Colorful Vegetables and Fruits: Recommend a variety of colorful vegetables and fruits rich in antioxidants, vitamins

and minerals to support overall health and hormonal stability.

6. Fermented Foods: Include fermented foods such as yogurt, kefir and sauerkraut, which contain probiotics that can help support gut health and indirectly influence hormonal balance.

7. Seeds: Suggest incorporating seeds such as flaxseeds, chia seeds and pumpkin seeds, which are rich in omega-3 fatty acids and lignans that can help promote hormonal stability.

8. Herbal Teas: Highlight the benefits of herbal teas such as green tea, chamomile and peppermint, which can have calming effects and support overall hormonal balance.

By incorporating these hormone-stabilizing foods into their diet, individuals can support their hormonal health and overall well-being following a hysterectomy. It's essential to consult with healthcare providers for personalized advice and guidance based on individual needs and circumstances.

9. OVERCOMING DIGESTIVE CHALLENGES

Overcoming digestive challenges is essential during the recovery period after a hysterectomy. Consider including the following tips and dietary recommendations in your cookbook to help readers manage digestive issues effectively:

1. Fiber-Rich Foods: Encourage the consumption of easily digestible fiber-rich foods such as cooked vegetables, ripe fruits and well-cooked grains to support healthy digestion without causing discomfort.

2. Probiotic-Rich Foods: Suggest incorporating probiotic-rich foods such as yogurt, kefir and fermented vegetables to promote a healthy gut microbiome and improve digestive function.

3. Hydration: Stress the importance of staying well-hydrated with water, herbal teas and clear broths to support digestion and prevent constipation during the recovery period.

4. Small, Frequent Meals: Encourage consuming small, frequent meals throughout the day rather than large, heavy meals to ease the digestive process and minimize discomfort.

5. Gentle Cooking Techniques: Recommend using gentle cooking techniques such as steaming, boiling and baking to prepare easily digestible meals and minimize digestive stress.

6. Avoiding Trigger Foods: Suggest avoiding spicy, greasy and heavily processed foods that may exacerbate digestive issues and cause discomfort during the recovery period.

7. Mindful Eating: Encourage mindful eating practices such as chewing food slowly, avoiding distractions and paying attention to hunger and fullness cues to support optimal digestion.

8. Consultation with Healthcare Providers: Stress the importance of consulting healthcare providers, including gastroenterologists or dietitians, to address specific digestive concerns and receive personalized guidance and support.

By incorporating these strategies into their daily routines, individuals can potentially overcome digestive challenges more effectively and support their overall well-being during the recovery period post-hysterectomy.

Foods to Aid Digestion and Bowel Movements

Including foods that aid digestion and promote regular bowel movements can be beneficial during the recovery period after a hysterectomy. Consider adding the following digestion-friendly foods and dietary recommendations to your cookbook:

1. Fiber-Rich Fruits: Encourage the consumption of easily digestible fruits such as ripe bananas, applesauce and berries, which can help promote healthy bowel movements and aid digestion.

2. Cooked Vegetables: Suggest incorporating well-cooked and easily digestible vegetables such as carrots, spinach and zucchini, which can provide essential nutrients while supporting digestive health.

3. Whole Grains: Include easily digestible whole grains such as oatmeal, white rice and quinoa, which can provide fiber to aid digestion and support regular bowel movements.

4. Probiotic-Rich Foods: Recommend incorporating probiotic-rich foods such as yogurt, kefir and kombucha, which can support a healthy gut microbiome and aid in digestion.

5. Healthy Fats: Suggest incorporating sources of healthy fats such as avocado, olive oil and nuts, which can support digestion and bowel regularity while providing essential nutrients.

6. Hydration: Stress the importance of staying well-hydrated with water, herbal teas and clear broths to promote optimal digestion and prevent constipation during the recovery period.

7. Herbal Teas: Include gentle and soothing herbal teas such as ginger, peppermint and chamomile, which can help alleviate digestive discomfort and promote healthy bowel movements.

8. Small, Frequent Meals: Encourage consuming small, frequent meals throughout the day to support digestion and minimize discomfort, allowing the digestive system to process food more efficiently.

By incorporating these digestion-friendly foods and dietary recommendations, individuals can support their digestive health and promote regular bowel movements during the recovery period post-hysterectomy. It's important to consult with healthcare providers for personalized advice and guidance based on individual needs and circumstances.

Balancing Fiber Intake

Balancing fiber intake is important for supporting digestive health and overall well-being, particularly during the recovery period after a hysterectomy. Consider including the following tips and dietary recommendations in your cookbook to help readers maintain a healthy balance of dietary fiber:

1. Gradual Increase: Encourage a gradual increase in fiber intake to allow the digestive system to adjust slowly, minimizing the risk of discomfort or digestive distress.

2. Fiber-Rich Fruits: Suggest incorporating a variety of fiber-rich fruits such as apples, pears and berries, which provide essential nutrients and promote digestive health.

3. Vegetables with Digestible Fiber: Include easily digestible vegetables such as cooked carrots, squash and green beans, which can provide fiber without causing digestive discomfort.

4. Whole Grains in Moderation: Recommend consuming whole grains such as brown rice, quinoa and oats in moderation to support a balanced fiber intake without overwhelming the digestive system.

5. Hydration: Emphasize the importance of staying well-hydrated with water, herbal teas and clear broths to support the effective movement of fiber through the digestive system and prevent constipation.

6. Probiotic Foods: Suggest incorporating probiotic-rich foods such as yogurt, kefir and kimchi to help maintain a healthy gut microbiome and support digestive balance when consuming fiber-rich foods.

7. Balanced Meals: Encourage the consumption of balanced meals that incorporate a mix of fiber, lean proteins and healthy fats to support overall digestion and promote sustained energy levels.

8. Mindful Portion Control: Stress the significance of mindful portion control to avoid excessive fiber intake, as overconsumption may lead to bloating, gas, or other digestive discomforts.

By incorporating these strategies into their daily routine, individuals can maintain a healthy balance of fiber intake and support their digestive health during the recovery period post-hysterectomy. It's important to consult with healthcare providers for personalized advice and guidance based on individual needs and circumstances.

10. LONG-TERM WELLNESS AND DIET

Promoting long-term wellness and a balanced diet is crucial for individuals post-hysterectomy. Consider including the following tips and dietary recommendations in your cookbook to help readers maintain a healthy lifestyle and overall well-being in the long term:

1. Whole Foods Emphasis: Encourage the consumption of whole, unprocessed foods such as fruits, vegetables, whole grains, lean proteins and healthy fats to provide essential nutrients and support overall health.

2. Moderation and Portion Control: Stress the importance of practicing moderation and portion control to maintain a healthy weight and support overall well-being without depriving oneself of favorite foods.

3. Regular Physical Activity: Emphasize the significance of engaging in regular physical activity, such as walking, jogging, yoga, or strength training, to support cardiovascular health, muscle strength and overall well-being.

4. Hydration: Highlight the importance of staying well-hydrated with water, herbal teas and hydrating foods to support overall health, digestion and the efficient functioning of bodily systems.

5. Mindful Eating Practices: Encourage the practice of mindful eating, including being aware of hunger and fullness cues, savoring each bite and focusing on the enjoyment and nourishment that food provides.

6. Stress Management Techniques: Suggest incorporating stress-reducing activities such as meditation, deep breathing exercises and hobbies to support emotional well-being and overall long-term health.

7. Regular Health Checkups: Stress the importance of regular health checkups and screenings to monitor overall health, address any potential concerns and receive personalized guidance for maintaining long-term wellness.

8. Variety and Balance: Encourage a diverse and balanced diet that includes a variety of nutrients, flavors and textures to ensure the body receives a wide array of essential vitamins and minerals for optimal health.

By incorporating these long-term wellness and dietary recommendations into their lifestyle, individuals can support their overall well-being and maintain a healthy and balanced approach to nutrition and health in the years following a hysterectomy.

Maintaining a Healthy Weight

Maintaining a healthy weight is essential for overall well-being, particularly following a hysterectomy. Consider including the following tips and dietary recommendations in your cookbook to help readers manage their weight effectively:

1. Balanced Meals: Encourage the consumption of balanced meals that include a mix of lean proteins, whole grains, healthy fats and a variety of fruits and vegetables to support satiety and overall health.

2. Portion Control: Stress the importance of mindful portion control to prevent overeating and support weight management, allowing individuals to enjoy a variety of foods without consuming excess calories.

3. Regular Physical Activity: Highlight the significance of engaging in regular physical activity, such as brisk walking, cycling, or swimming, to support calorie expenditure, muscle strength and overall well-being.

4. Healthy Snacking: Suggest incorporating healthy snacks such as nuts, fruits and yogurt to support energy levels and prevent overeating during main meals, promoting better weight management.

5. Hydration: Emphasize the importance of staying well-hydrated with water and herbal teas, as adequate hydration can support metabolism and help individuals differentiate between hunger and thirst cues.

6. Mindful Eating Practices: Encourage the practice of mindful eating, which involves paying attention to hunger and fullness cues, eating slowly and savoring each bite to prevent overeating and support weight management.

7. Limiting Sugary and Processed Foods: Stress the significance of minimizing the intake of sugary beverages, processed snacks and high-calorie desserts to reduce overall calorie intake and support weight management.

8. Regular Health Checkups: Encourage regular health checkups to monitor weight and receive personalized guidance from healthcare providers to maintain a healthy weight and overall well-being.

By incorporating these strategies into their lifestyle, individuals can effectively manage their weight and support their overall well-being following a hysterectomy. It's essential to consult with healthcare providers for personalized advice and guidance based on individual needs and circumstances.

Sustainable Eating Habits Post-Recovery

Promoting sustainable eating habits post-recovery is essential for long-term well-being and overall health. Consider including the following tips and dietary recommendations in your cookbook to help readers maintain sustainable and healthy eating habits:

1. Seasonal and Local Produce: Encourage the consumption of seasonal and locally sourced fruits and vegetables to support sustainable food choices and reduce the carbon footprint.

2. Plant-Based Meals: Suggest incorporating more plant-based meals into the diet, such as legumes, whole grains and a variety of vegetables, to promote sustainable eating habits and support overall health.

3. Reducing Food Waste: Stress the importance of minimizing food waste by planning meals, utilizing leftovers and storing food properly to support sustainable practices and reduce environmental impact.

4. Mindful Consumption: Encourage mindful consumption by being aware of portion sizes, choosing nutrient-dense foods and savoring each bite to promote sustainable eating habits and prevent overconsumption.

5. Sustainable Protein Sources: Highlight the benefits of incorporating sustainable protein sources such as legumes, tofu and responsibly sourced seafood to support sustainable eating habits and reduce environmental impact.

6. Reducing Processed Foods: Stress the significance of minimizing the intake of processed and packaged foods to promote sustainable eating habits and support overall health and well-being.

7. Hydration with Sustainable Options: Encourage the consumption of sustainably sourced water and herbal teas, as well as reducing the use of single-use plastic bottles, to promote sustainable hydration practices.

8. Educational Resources: Provide educational resources on sustainable eating practices, such as information on local farmers' markets, community-supported agriculture (CSA) programs and sustainable food certifications, to support informed and sustainable food choices.

By incorporating these sustainable eating habits into their lifestyle, individuals can contribute to a healthier and more environmentally friendly food system while supporting their long-term well-being and overall health following a hysterectomy.

11. PSYCHOLOGICAL WELL-BEING AND FOOD

Promoting psychological well-being through food can play a significant role in supporting overall mental health and emotional resilience, particularly during the recovery period after a hysterectomy. Consider including the following tips and dietary recommendations in your cookbook to help readers foster a positive relationship with food and support their psychological well-being:

1. Mood-Boosting Foods: Suggest incorporating mood-boosting foods such as dark chocolate, berries and nuts, which contain antioxidants and compounds that may positively influence mood and emotional well-being.

2. Comforting and Nourishing Meals: Offer recipes for comforting and nourishing meals that evoke positive emotions and provide a sense of warmth and comfort, supporting psychological well-being during the recovery process.

3. Mindful Eating Practices: Emphasize the practice of mindful eating, which involves paying attention to the sensory experience of eating, fostering a healthy relationship with food and promoting positive emotional connections with meals.

4. Social Dining: Encourage social dining experiences with friends and family to foster a sense of connection and support, promoting positive emotional well-being and enhancing the overall dining experience.

5. Supportive Nutrition Education: Provide educational resources on the connection between food and mood, emphasizing the importance of nutrient-dense foods and balanced meals in supporting overall psychological well-being.

6. Incorporating Variety: Encourage the incorporation of a variety of flavors, textures and colors in meals to stimulate the senses and promote a positive and enjoyable dining experience, supporting emotional well-being.

7. Stress-Reducing Nutrients: Highlight the benefits of incorporating stress-reducing nutrients such as omega-3 fatty acids, B vitamins and magnesium, which can help support emotional resilience and overall psychological well-being.

8. Culinary Therapy: Suggest engaging in culinary activities such as cooking, baking and food styling, which can serve as a form of therapeutic expression and provide a sense of accomplishment and joy.

By incorporating these psychological well-being-focused dietary recommendations into their cookbook, readers can foster a positive relationship with food and support their emotional resilience and overall well-being during the recovery period post-hysterectomy.

Foods for Mood and Stress Management

Incorporating foods that support mood and stress management can be beneficial for individuals during the recovery period after a hysterectomy. Consider including the following mood-boosting and stress-reducing foods and dietary recommendations in your cookbook:

1. Complex Carbohydrates: Encourage the consumption of complex carbohydrates such as whole grains, sweet potatoes and oats, which can help regulate serotonin levels and promote a sense of calm and well-being.

2. Fatty Fish: Include fatty fish such as salmon, mackerel and trout, which are rich in omega-3 fatty acids that can help reduce inflammation and support brain health, potentially improving mood and reducing stress.

3. Leafy Greens: Suggest incorporating leafy greens like spinach, kale and Swiss chard, which are rich in folate and magnesium, supporting the production of mood-regulating neurotransmitters and aiding in stress management.

4. Nuts and Seeds: Highlight the benefits of consuming nuts and seeds such as almonds, walnuts and sunflower seeds, which contain stress-reducing nutrients like magnesium, zinc and B vitamins.

5. Berries: Encourage the consumption of antioxidant-rich berries such as blueberries, strawberries and raspberries, which can help combat oxidative stress and support overall brain health and mood regulation.

6. Probiotic-Rich Foods: Suggest incorporating probiotic-rich foods such as yogurt, kefir and kimchi, which can support gut health and potentially improve mood and stress resilience.

7. Dark Chocolate: Include moderate amounts of dark chocolate, which contains flavonoids that can help reduce stress hormones and promote the release of endorphins, contributing to a sense of well-being and relaxation.

8. Herbal Teas: Recommend soothing herbal teas such as chamomile, lavender and lemon balm, which can have calming effects and promote relaxation and stress reduction.

By incorporating these mood-boosting and stress-reducing foods into their diet, individuals can support their emotional well-being and stress management during the recovery period post-hysterectomy. It's important to consult with healthcare providers for personalized advice and guidance based on individual needs and circumstances.

Self-care and Mindful Eating Tips

Promoting self-care and mindful eating practices can contribute to overall well-being and support individuals during the recovery period after a hysterectomy. Consider including the following self-care and mindful eating tips in your cookbook to help readers foster a positive relationship with food and support their emotional and physical well-being:

1. Setting the Right Environment: Encourage creating a peaceful and inviting dining environment that promotes relaxation and enjoyment during meal times, fostering a positive and mindful eating experience.

2. Mindful Meal Preparation: Suggest engaging in mindful meal preparation, including selecting fresh ingredients, practicing gratitude for the nourishment provided and savoring the process of cooking, to cultivate a sense of mindfulness and self-care.

3. Mindful Eating Techniques: Emphasize the practice of mindful eating techniques such as chewing slowly, savoring each bite and paying attention to hunger and fullness cues to promote a deeper connection with food and enhance the overall dining experience.

4. Portion Awareness: Stress the importance of being aware of portion sizes and practicing portion control to support balanced eating habits and prevent overeating, fostering a mindful approach to food consumption.

5. Emotional Check-Ins: Encourage individuals to check in with their emotions before and after eating, allowing them to recognize any emotional triggers related to food and develop healthier coping mechanisms that support emotional well-being.

6. Gratitude Practice: Suggest incorporating a gratitude practice before meals, acknowledging the efforts involved in meal preparation and expressing gratitude for the nourishment provided, fostering a sense of appreciation and well-being.

7. Sensory Engagement: Highlight the importance of engaging the senses while eating, including appreciating the aroma, texture and flavors of the food, to promote a more profound and mindful connection with the dining experience.

8. Reflective Journaling: Encourage reflective journaling about the eating experience, including thoughts and feelings related to food choices and the overall dining

experience, fostering self-awareness and promoting emotional well-being.

By incorporating these self-care and mindful eating tips into their daily routine, individuals can foster a positive relationship with food and support their emotional and physical well-being during the recovery period post-hysterectomy.

12. RECIPES FOR SUSTAINABLE HEALTH

Certainly! Here are a few recipes for sustainable health that you can consider including in your cookbook:

1. Quinoa and Chickpea Salad:

   - Ingredients: Quinoa, chickpeas, cherry tomatoes, cucumber, fresh parsley, lemon juice, olive oil, salt and pepper.

   - Instructions: Cook quinoa according to package instructions. Mix quinoa with chickpeas, cherry tomatoes and cucumber. Add fresh parsley, lemon juice, olive oil, salt and pepper to taste. Toss well and serve.

2. Stuffed Bell Peppers with Lentils:

   - Ingredients: Bell peppers, lentils, onion, garlic, spinach, tomato sauce, paprika, cumin, salt and pepper.

   - Instructions: Preheat oven to 375°F. Cook lentils according to package instructions. Sauté onion and garlic, then add spinach and cooked lentils. Season with paprika, cumin, salt and pepper. Stuff the bell peppers with the lentil mixture and bake for 25-30 minutes.

3. Roasted Vegetable Buddha Bowl:

   - Ingredients: Sweet potatoes, Brussels sprouts, broccoli, chickpeas, quinoa, tahini, lemon juice, olive oil, salt and pepper.

- Instructions: Preheat oven to 400°F. Toss sweet potatoes, Brussels sprouts and broccoli with olive oil, salt and pepper. Roast for 25-30 minutes. Prepare quinoa according to package instructions. Assemble the bowl with quinoa, roasted vegetables and chickpeas. Drizzle with tahini and lemon juice.

4. Vegan Lentil Curry:

  - Ingredients: Lentils, coconut milk, curry paste, onion, garlic, ginger, carrots, spinach, turmeric, cumin, salt and pepper.

  - Instructions: Cook lentils according to package instructions. Sauté onion, garlic and ginger. Add carrots and spinach. Stir in curry paste, turmeric and cumin. Pour in coconut milk and cooked lentils. Simmer for 15-20 minutes.

5. Berry and Oatmeal Breakfast Smoothie:

  - Ingredients: Mixed berries, rolled oats, banana, spinach, almond milk, chia seeds and honey (optional).

  - Instructions: Blend mixed berries, rolled oats, banana, spinach, almond milk and chia seeds until smooth. Add honey for sweetness if desired. Serve chilled.

These recipes prioritize the use of sustainable ingredients and offer a balance of essential nutrients for a wholesome and nourishing meal experience.

Nourishing and Delicious Meal Plans

Certainly! Here are a few nourishing and delicious meal plans that you can consider including in your cookbook:

Day 1:

- Breakfast: Mixed Berry and Yogurt Parfait with Granola.

- Lunch: Quinoa Salad with Roasted Vegetables and Lemon-Tahini Dressing.

- Dinner: Baked Salmon with Steamed Asparagus and Herbed Brown Rice.

Day 2:

- Breakfast: Spinach and Mushroom Omelette with Whole Grain Toast.

- Lunch: Lentil Soup with a Side of Mixed Green Salad.

- Dinner: Grilled Chicken Breast with Sautéed Zucchini and Wild Rice Pilaf.

Day 3:

- Breakfast: Overnight Chia Seed Pudding with Fresh Fruit and Almonds.

- Lunch: Chickpea and Avocado Salad with Lemon Vinaigrette.

- Dinner: Vegetable Stir-Fry with Tofu and Brown Rice.

Day 4:

- Breakfast: Oatmeal with Sliced Banana and a Drizzle of Honey.

- Lunch: Mediterranean Quinoa Bowl with Hummus and Falafel.

- Dinner: Turkey Meatballs with Marinara Sauce over Whole Wheat Spaghetti.

Day 5:

- Breakfast: Whole Grain Pancakes with Mixed Berries and Maple Syrup.

- Lunch: Black Bean and Corn Salad with Cilantro-Lime Dressing.

- Dinner: Baked Cod with Roasted Brussels Sprouts and Garlic Mashed Potatoes.

Reintroducing Regular Foods Safely

Reintroducing regular foods safely after a period of dietary restrictions is crucial for individuals recovering from a medical procedure such as a hysterectomy. Here are some tips you can include in your cookbook:

1. Start Slowly: Begin reintroducing regular foods gradually, starting with small portions to assess how your body reacts to different food groups.

2. Monitor Symptoms: Keep a food journal to track any adverse reactions or digestive issues that may occur when reintroducing specific foods, helping to identify potential triggers.

3. Choose Easily Digestible Foods: Opt for easily digestible foods such as cooked vegetables, lean proteins and whole grains to reintroduce regular foods while minimizing digestive discomfort.

4. Avoid Trigger Foods: Steer clear of foods that were problematic before the surgery or during the recovery period, as they may still cause digestive issues when reintroduced.

5. Consult a Healthcare Professional: Seek guidance from a healthcare provider or a registered dietitian who can provide personalized recommendations and monitor your progress as you reintroduce regular foods.

6. Balanced Diet: Focus on maintaining a balanced diet that includes a variety of nutrient-dense foods to ensure you are getting the necessary vitamins and minerals while reintroducing regular foods.

7. Hydration: Stay well-hydrated by drinking an adequate amount of water throughout the day, as it can help support digestion and overall well-being during the reintroduction process.

8. Patience and Observation: Be patient with the process of reintroducing regular foods and be attentive to how your body responds, adjusting your diet accordingly to promote optimal digestion and overall health.

By incorporating these tips into your cookbook, you can provide valuable guidance for individuals navigating the reintroduction of regular foods after a period of dietary restrictions, supporting a safe and smooth transition to a balanced and varied diet.

13. FREQUENTLY ASKED QUESTIONS

Common Concerns and Queries Answered

Addressing common concerns and queries in your cookbook can provide valuable information and support for individuals during their recovery from a hysterectomy. Consider including answers to the following common concerns and queries:

1. Physical Activity: Discuss the appropriate timeline for resuming physical activity and exercise post-hysterectomy, emphasizing the importance of starting slowly and gradually increasing intensity.

2. Medication Management: Provide guidance on managing pain and discomfort with prescribed medications, including potential side effects and interactions to watch for.

3. Follow-Up Care: Explain the importance of regular follow-up appointments with healthcare providers, highlighting the significance of monitoring recovery progress and addressing any concerns or complications.

4. Emotional Support: Offer resources and tips for seeking emotional support, such as joining support groups, talking to a therapist, or engaging in stress-relieving activities to manage emotional challenges during the recovery period.

5. Scar Management: Provide suggestions for scar management, including proper wound care, use of scar-reducing creams and gentle massage techniques to promote healing and minimize scarring.

6. Sleep and Rest: Discuss the significance of adequate sleep and rest in the recovery process, offering tips for creating a comfortable sleep environment and practicing relaxation techniques to promote quality sleep.

7. Resuming Daily Activities: Offer guidance on gradually resuming daily activities, such as lifting, driving and household chores, emphasizing the importance of listening to the body and avoiding overexertion during the recovery period.

8. Dietary Adjustments: Explain any necessary dietary adjustments, such as managing fiber intake, staying hydrated and incorporating nutrient-dense foods to support the body's healing process and overall well-being.

By addressing these common concerns and queries in your cookbook, you can provide individuals with comprehensive information and guidance, empowering them to navigate the recovery process with confidence and support.

Professional Guidance and Support

Emphasizing the importance of seeking professional guidance and support during the recovery process is crucial in your cookbook. Here are some key points to highlight:

1. Healthcare Providers: Encourage readers to maintain regular communication with their healthcare providers, including surgeons, gynecologists and primary care physicians, to receive professional guidance and support tailored to their specific recovery needs.

2. Registered Dietitians: Stress the importance of consulting registered dietitians to create personalized meal plans that address individual dietary requirements and promote optimal healing and well-being.

3. Physical Therapists: Highlight the role of physical therapists in guiding individuals through tailored exercise programs that promote safe and effective rehabilitation, helping to restore strength and mobility after surgery.

4. Mental Health Professionals: Encourage individuals to seek support from mental health professionals, such as counselors or therapists, to address any emotional challenges or psychological concerns that may arise during the recovery process.

5. Support Groups: Suggest the benefits of joining support groups or online communities where individuals can connect with others who have undergone similar procedures, fostering a sense of camaraderie and providing emotional support and encouragement.

6. Home Care Providers: Acknowledge the assistance of home care providers or caregivers in facilitating a smooth recovery process, especially for individuals who may require additional help with daily activities and tasks.

7. Rehabilitation Centers: Provide information on rehabilitation centers or specialized facilities that offer comprehensive post-surgery rehabilitation programs, including physical therapy, occupational therapy and other supportive services.

By emphasizing the significance of seeking professional guidance and support, you can empower individuals to prioritize their well-being and recovery journey, ensuring they have access to the necessary resources and assistance needed to promote a successful and effective recovery process after a hysterectomy.

14. CONCLUSION

Embracing a New Chapter of Health

Encouraging individuals to embrace a new chapter of health post-hysterectomy can provide them with the motivation and confidence needed to embark on their journey toward well-being. Here are some suggestions to include in your cookbook:

1. Positive Affirmations: Integrate positive affirmations and motivational messages that inspire readers to embrace the opportunity for improved health and well-being, fostering a sense of optimism and resilience.

2. Goal Setting: Encourage individuals to set realistic and achievable health goals, such as incorporating regular physical activity, maintaining a balanced diet and practicing self-care, to promote a proactive and empowered approach to their well-being.

3. Mind-Body Connection: Stress the importance of nurturing the mind-body connection through practices such as meditation, mindfulness and relaxation techniques, promoting holistic wellness and emotional balance.

4. Adaptive Strategies: Provide adaptive strategies and resources that support individuals in adjusting to potential

physical and emotional changes, empowering them to adapt and thrive in their new chapter of health.

5. Celebrating Progress: Encourage celebrating each milestone and achievement along the journey toward improved health, fostering a sense of accomplishment and motivation to continue making positive lifestyle choices.

6. Community Engagement: Highlight the benefits of engaging with a supportive community, whether through local groups, online forums, or social networks, fostering a sense of belonging and shared experiences that can inspire and uplift individuals.

7. Continual Learning: Promote the importance of ongoing learning and self-improvement in the realm of health and wellness, encouraging individuals to stay informed and curious about new developments and practices that can further enhance their well-being.

By incorporating these suggestions into your cookbook, you can inspire individuals to embrace their new chapter of health with confidence and enthusiasm, fostering a positive and proactive approach to their overall well-being post-hysterectomy.

Lasting Dietary Principles for Well-being

Encouraging lasting dietary principles for overall well-being can help individuals maintain a healthy and balanced lifestyle beyond the recovery period post-hysterectomy. Here are some key dietary principles to include in your cookbook:

1. Whole Foods Emphasis: Promote the consumption of whole, minimally processed foods such as fruits, vegetables, whole grains, lean proteins and healthy fats to ensure a nutrient-rich diet.

2. Moderation and Balance: Stress the importance of practicing moderation and balance when it comes to portion sizes and food choices to support a sustainable and enjoyable approach to eating.

3. Hydration: Emphasize the significance of staying well-hydrated by drinking an adequate amount of water throughout the day to support overall health and bodily functions.

4. Mindful Eating Practices: Encourage mindful eating habits, including slowing down during meals, savoring the flavors and textures of food and paying attention to hunger and fullness cues to promote a healthier relationship with food.

5. Diverse Nutrient Intake: Encourage individuals to consume a diverse range of nutrients from various food groups, ensuring they receive a wide array of vitamins, minerals and antioxidants that are essential for overall well-being.

6. Personalized Meal Planning: Advocate for personalized meal planning based on individual dietary needs, preferences and any specific health considerations, ensuring a tailored approach to nutrition and well-being.

7. Sustainable Choices: Promote making sustainable food choices, including selecting locally sourced and seasonal produce, supporting sustainable farming practices and minimizing food waste to promote environmental well-being.

8. Lifelong Learning: Encourage individuals to stay informed and continue learning about nutrition, health and wellness, enabling them to make informed and empowered choices that support their long-term well-being.

By integrating these lasting dietary principles into your cookbook, you can empower individuals to adopt a sustainable and holistic approach to their dietary habits, supporting their overall well-being and long-term health post-hysterectomy.

15. Appendix

Additional Resources and References

Incorporating additional resources and references in your cookbook can provide individuals with a comprehensive source of information and support as they navigate their recovery journey post-hysterectomy. Consider including the following:

1. Scientific Journals: List reputable scientific journals in the fields of nutrition, women's health and surgery that publish research related to dietary considerations and recovery guidelines for individuals undergoing a hysterectomy.

2. Nutritional Guidelines: Include references to official nutritional guidelines from renowned organizations such as the World Health Organization (WHO), the Academy of Nutrition and Dietetics and the American College of Obstetricians and Gynecologists (ACOG) that offer evidence-based recommendations for post-operative nutrition.

3. Clinical Studies: Cite relevant clinical studies and research papers that investigate the impact of dietary interventions on post-surgical recovery, emphasizing findings that

support specific dietary recommendations and best practices for individuals following a hysterectomy.

4. Patient Support Organizations: Provide information on reputable patient support organizations and foundations dedicated to women's health, surgery recovery and holistic well-being, offering individuals access to a network of resources, educational materials and community support.

5. Medical Literature Reviews: Refer to medical literature reviews that summarize current knowledge and advancements in the field of gynecological surgery, highlighting key insights into post-operative care, nutritional support and long-term wellness considerations for individuals recovering from a hysterectomy.

6. Government Health Agencies: Direct readers to government health agencies such as the Centers for Disease Control and Prevention (CDC) and the National Institutes of Health (NIH), which offer comprehensive health information and resources on post-operative care and dietary guidelines for women undergoing surgical procedures.

7. Patient Education Materials: Include patient education materials provided by reputable healthcare institutions, surgical centers and women's health clinics, offering

practical tips, dietary recommendations and lifestyle guidance tailored to individuals recovering from a hysterectomy.

By incorporating these additional resources and references, you can provide individuals with a well-rounded and informative resource that supports their recovery journey and empowers them to make informed decisions about their dietary and wellness needs post-hysterectomy.

Further Reading and Support

Including recommendations for further reading and support in your cookbook can provide individuals with additional resources and guidance to continue their journey toward improved health and well-being. Consider suggesting the following:

1. Books on Nutrition and Wellness: Recommend reputable books that focus on nutrition, healthy eating and overall wellness, providing valuable insights and practical tips for maintaining a balanced and nourishing diet.

2. Online Resources: Suggest reliable websites, blogs and online platforms that offer evidence-based information on health, nutrition and lifestyle, empowering individuals to access a wealth of knowledge and support at their convenience.

3. Support Groups: Provide information on local or online support groups specifically tailored to individuals who have undergone a hysterectomy, fostering a sense of community and offering a platform for sharing experiences and receiving mutual support.

4. Professional Associations: Encourage individuals to explore professional associations related to nutrition, dietetics and women's health, where they can access expert

guidance, research updates and educational materials from reputable professionals in the field.

5. Health and Wellness Workshops: Highlight the benefits of attending health and wellness workshops, seminars and webinars that focus on various aspects of well-being, providing opportunities for individuals to learn from experts and engage in interactive discussions on relevant topics.

6. Counseling Services: Recommend seeking counseling services or mental health support for individuals who may need additional guidance in coping with emotional challenges or psychological adjustments following a significant medical procedure.

7. Community Resources: Provide information on community resources such as local health clinics, women's health centers and wellness programs that offer a range of services, including nutritional counseling, exercise classes and holistic wellness initiatives.

By offering these suggestions for further reading and support, you can equip individuals with the tools and resources needed to continue their journey toward improved health and well-being, ensuring they have access to a supportive network and valuable information as they navigate life post-hysterectomy.